Diabetes and Heart Diseases

What the Doctor will not tell you

K. Raveendran

ISBN-10: 1987723732

ISBN-13: 978-1987723731

Table of Contents

About this Book

I have written this Book for sharing my experience for the benefit of millions of people who are suffering from diabetes and related problems like cardio vascular diseases, diabetic retinopathy, kidney failure, and liver related problems such as Fatty Liver, Gall bladder stones etc. Like the saying goes, prevention is better than cure, there is no better way than preventing the problems at the early stage through judicious use of food, medicine and exercises. So that it will not grow into a chronic case and that will save you huge amount of money, relief from related side effects and avoid inconvenience to your family.

Myself is a diabetic patient for over 25 years, aged 60 years and has undergone a bypass surgery (CABG) and mitral valve replacement surgery (MVR) simultaneously in 2015. I hope the information (such as need for exercise, total and strict control over your diet, proper and timely medication) provided in this Book will be of immense help to people who are suffering from diabetes, cardio vascular diseases and other problems. It may also be of immense help or may be of use as a guide to individuals in whose home or in their family, there is someone who is suffering from diabetes and other related diseases.

I have tried to include every aspect of the problems in a simple way viz selection of food especially type of foods that you have to consume to bring down your glucose level. How you can prevent various problems such as blood pressure, obesity, fatty liver etc. by adopting healthy foods in your daily consumption, regular exercise, and medication. I will also show you how I reduced my HbA1c or the Estimated Glucose level from 6.8 i.e controlled diabetes to 5.7 i.e. pre-diabetic level through strict control over diet in just five months of adoption of them. Hope you will enjoy reading this Book, follow the tips given herein, and adopt it in your daily life so that you can enjoy life and be worry free.

Chapter 1

Introduction

According to World Health Organization, over 422 million   (as of 2014 data which is growing at a rate of 9.3% currently) people are suffering from Diabetes and over 17.7 million people died in 2015 due to Cardio Vascular Diseases,   of which 6.7 million deaths were due to stroke. Many a times it has been found that both the diseases are caused more by lifestyle related problems than any other causes. Sometimes, diabetes can be hereditary or genetic related. If you are a diabetic and the blood sugar levels are not controlled, then you are 100% sure to have other problems related to heart, kidney, and liver.

Out of these, heart ailments are the most common disease faced by diabetic patient's viz. coronary artery disease, mitral and/or aortic valve problems, high cholesterol, depression, and obesity. All these are life threatening, and to be diagnosed and treated early. Worldwide the cost of CVD was $ 863 billion in 2010, and projected to be a whooping $1044 billion by the year 2030.

You may be wondering what this person is writing about. He is neither a doctor nor an expert in medical field. I have undergone a bypass surgery and mitral valve replacement surgery simultaneously, lasting over nine hours in February 2015.

Again, two major eye surgeries viz Vitrectomy (retinal surgery) of the right eye in January 2016 and a Vitreous Lavage surgery (known as washing of the retina) in November 2016 due to Diabetic Retinopathy and Vitreous Hemorrhage (internal bleeding in the eye). Thereafter in February 2018, a cataract surgery of the same eye as well.

However, the problem of bleeding from both the eyes intermittently in the gap of every 4-6 months have been continuing and not stopped so far. When one stops, the other starts and so on. The bleeding, which started after five months of my MV replacement surgery, is induced by Acitrom, a tablet which I take for the health of my mechanical heart valve.

I have been active, not very slim, or over weight, no drinking or smoking habits, and do general exercises, taking medication and generally adhering to my diets.

The only thing that I did not follow was strictly adhering to a diet plan.

Many diabetic consultants or small hospitals do not have a dietician in the clinic or hospital, except big corporate hospital, that too only with a Cardiologist and not with endocrinologist or the so-called diabetic specialist. However, in Government Medical Colleges, you will find at least one dietician.

The qualities of most of these dieticians are very poor as they get very low salaries as such casual in approach.

Interestingly, I do not have any of the major symptoms of diabetes viz. frequent urination, perspiration, extreme thirst, and hunger. Perhaps this may be due to DNA problem, which can only diagnosed with a DNA or genetic Assay. A DNA test is very costly and many doctors do not recommend it.

I wish to share the important experience of mine, for the benefit of all diabetic, heart, eye, kidney, and liver patients. Take appropriate corrective steps to prevent all the problems that I have gone through and save you from these chronic diseases and save money, avoid hospitalization, enjoy life and difficulties to your near and dear.

As all of you know, diabetics, especially the type two patients i.e. insulin dependent adults over 50 years, both men and women are more prone to heart diseases. Unlike other patients, heart patients who already have a history of diabetes face a situation, where he/she will not even know that you have heart problems, until it is too late as there will not be any signals. It spreads silently from one organ to the other. Therefore, you have to be extremely cautious and alert to avoid emergent situations.

Other long-term complications of diabetes are vision problems, kidney failure, liver complications like Fatty liver, Liver Cirrhosis, and sometimes - liver cancer. This condition is not diagnosed and treated early can lead to surgery or even liver transplantation, which is too costly.

Chapter 2

Diabetes

Everybody knows that diabetes is the problem of high sugar or glucose levels in the body. However to define diabetes, you must understand what exactly it is. When you eat food, the organ called pancreas produce insulin, which is the key to open the cells in your body and then only the body will absorb the sugar or glucose obtained from the food.

The food converted into sugar or glucose contain essential nutrients, minerals, carbohydrates and antioxidants which gives energy, immunity and helps in body growth. When your body does not produce sufficient quantity of insulin, the glucose or sugar levels goes up and the essential nutrients may not reach inside the cells. This is diabetes.

Symptoms of Diabetes

Excessive thirst, hunger, perspiration, frequent urination and sudden vision change or blurring of vision, tingling, or numbness in feet or hand, feeling tired most of the time, dry skin, sores those are slow to heal, and more infections than usual are some of the symptoms of diabetes.

When your body did not produce the required quantity of insulin, you need medication through tablets and injections to control the raised glucose levels in the body. Generally, diabetes is a hereditary problem; however, lifestyle changes and diet habits can cause diabetes. Since this is a chronic disease, this cannot cure completely, but can control through right treatment.

When you go to a doctor for treatment of diabetes, the doctor prescribes a few tests and after analyzing the type of diabetes, he/she prescribes some medicines for BP, Sugar and gives you some pamphlets to read about the disease and to ensure that you become aware of the causes of the disease and follow instructions to prevent it.

However, in majority of cases, due to lack of time and the greed for money, it prevents them from giving you the right advice. They treat you as the golden egg laying hen as you will be a lifelong patient for him/her. There may be a few exceptions, but majority of doctors fall in this category.

Normally, the doctor advices a few tests viz, GTT (Glucose tolerance test), Lipid profile consisting of Triglycerides, HDL, LDL, and Total cholesterol. In addition, Fasting and post lunch blood sugar including urine sugar and complete urine examinations. SometimesHbA1c/eAG, estimated average glucose in mg/dl (a blood test to determine the stage of diabetes and/or to ascertain the estimated average glucose level in your body for the next three months, based on which the physician plans treatment.

If your HbA1c level is 5.5 (117 mg/dl or less), then you are not diabetic, but 6.5 to 7 (140 to 154 mg/dl) controlled diabetic and if your A1c level is 8, (183 mg/dl or more) then you are in danger and you may definitely have cardiac problems like CAD. Before surgery my A1c level was 10, then 9 and at the time of CABG surgery it was 8.5. However, after surgery, it is 6.8 and recently i.e. in February 2018, it has come down to 5.7 that means, to pre-diabetic stage.

Chapter 3

Related Problems of Diabetes

The major problems encountered by diabetic patients are Cardio Vascular Diseases, Kidney failure, Liver Diseases and Ophthalmic problems. The details of which are given below in brief.

Cardio Vascular Disease

Coronary artery disease (CAD) is one of the major side effects of diabetes, which spreads very slowly and silently, resulting in the blockage of arteries and thereby putting increased pressure on the blood vessels. Owing to this, you will not get fresh oxygen and nutrients in the required quantity and results in high blood pressure.

Other diseases are valvular disease, and cardio myopathy, which affect the heart muscles, heart rhythm and heart infections. The main cause of CVD is uncontrolled and prolonged diabetes in addition to life style and sometimes hereditary/ congenital problems.

Some of the main symptoms of heart attack is chest pain, which spread to the arm, neck, or back; sweating, shortness of breath and nausea.

Eye Disorders

Next comes eye related problems like Diabetic Retinopathy both non proliferative and proliferative, known as NPDR and PDR, including retinal damages, vitreous hemorrhage and sometimes partial or total loss of vision. This can lead to various ophthalmic problems   and need laser treatment and/or surgeries like, Vitrectomy, which may develop cataract immediately after surgery or within two years of surgery, vitreous lavage etc.

In my case, I have cataract within two months after surgery. Therefore, regular check up in a good eye hospital under qualified and reputed ophthalmologist is essential. The ideal interval for check up is once in every six months, and in the least case, once a year.

A small Tip

One of the retina physicians I met sometime in 2016 advised and reminded me that the moment I was detected with diabetes, could have started using insulin, instead of managing with tablets for a long time, as it will prevent further damages and could have controlled the diabetes. Not only this, use of insulin will give you overall better health.

Perhaps, the fear of pain from the insulin needles may be preventing you from going in for insulin injections, this was the case with me initially, but the small insulin needles like the small Novo fine needles are sharp and painless unlike the standard insulin syringe.

Therefore, my dear friends, if you have been suffering from diabetes from an early age, say from around 30 plus, then it is better to start using insulin, even if it is only 1 or 2 units daily or may be once in a week. This will save your life. However, consult your doctor first, and then only start using insulin, as self-mediation is dangerous.

Liver Diseases

Liver is an important organ in the body and when someone is having prolonged and uncontrolled diabetes, this vital organ can get damaged. The most common disease affecting liver is Fatty Liver and Liver Cirrhosis.

Normally the liver diseases is diagnosed with some of the tests like, Liver Function Test. Imaging tests like CT, MRI or ultrasound scanning and sometimes through a biopsy to ascertain the problem. Liver problems can be treated with medication, modifying life styles and in extreme cases by surgery and/or liver transplantation.

Kidney Disease

My dear friends, as you are aware, the most common cause of kidney failure is due to prolonged diabetes and hypertension. Some of the major symptoms of kidney failure are nausea, sleeping trouble, poor appetite, weakness or tiredness, itching, weight loss, muscle cramps, especially in the legs, pedal edema i.e. swelling in your feet or ankles, and anemia.

The main tests used to ascertain your kidneys health is ACR (Albumin to Creatinine Ratio) and eGFR (estimated Glomerular Function Rate) BP, Blood Sugar, and cholesterol levels. Doctors normally try medicinal treatments, but when in case of kidney failure, there are only two options, one is dialysis viz hemodialysis or peritoneal dialysis, and the other is kidney transplantation. In both the cases it is very costly. Therefore, it is better to take care of your kidneys well by controlling BP, and sugar through medicines, exercise, and life style modifications in order to save money, troubles, and life itself.

Note: Sometimes, some persons get kidney stones in their kidney(s), may be from foods, or sometimes from prolonged allopathic medications. Generally, if you drink lots of water, it will be washed away naturally. In case, it did not go and you have severe pain, then, it needs to be removed using non-surgical procedures or with a small surgery.

Obesity

Obesity is a condition in which the body accumulates fat and unused glucose, which will be harmful to your life. Normally, women and to some extent men fall prey to this problem. Women, especially, those who are home makers or go for work outside, are prone to obese conditions due to stressful life, and in certain conditions like, diabetes, and thyroid problems.

A body mass index above 30 is considered as obese and a BMI greater than 40 is classified as morbid obese. In such conditions, the patient irrespective of gender, need medical attention and treatment to control it or sometimes-surgical procedures are used.

However, all these categories of persons, male or female can reduce their weight, without spending too much money that spent on buying costly, and useless supplements and other scientifically untested and not proven medications. Instead buy the foods mentioned in this book, that is natural, wholesome and healthy. If you genuinely try to adhere to a plan, then you can definitely, reduce weight without pinching your pocket and be healthy. It can happen in a few months and over a year's use of the healthy foods like whole grains, fruits, and vegetables you will definitely become healthy and of normal weight. So go for it instead of wasting money on the so-called natural foods, in the name of supplements.

Chapter 4

What the doctor will not tell you

I have not come across any diabetic specialists advising patients to have a cardiac risk test in people over 45 and have prolonged treatment for diabetes. Generally, they will not advice you to undergo a TMT or CT Angiogram (CTA) test to ascertain whether you have any arterial blockages commonly called CAD.

The only exception is when you have so many problems related to heart; they will recommend you to a cardiologist for further specialist consultation and advice.

A 2D echo will reveal the condition of your heart, however, may not reveal blockages, but any problems with heart valves will definitely revealed.

Though an ECG reveals heart problems, a TMT or CT Angiogram test will reveal CAD. I feel that a CT Angiogram is the best test to know the exact percentage of blockages, if any, in the heart, which will save your time, money and tension as well. This test is done to know whether you have any blockages, then based on the results, the doctor advises actual Angiogram, which can be done only in the hospital as an inpatient.

My Experience

I am writing this from my own experience of taking treatment for diabetes for the past 25 years from different physicians specializing in diabetic treatment. This includes big corporate hospitals and super specialists called endocrinologists. Even the Cardiologists will not advice a CT Angiogram until the disease has reached a stage, which is ready for surgery.

They will give you the right doses of insulin, general diet control advice, various types of tablets to control high blood pressure, and allied problems. However, they will not tell you what exactly to be done to control your glucose levels except instructing you to increase the insulin dosages.

Suppose, you are admitted to the hospital due to high glucose levels or high BP, the doctor controls it within a few days with right doses of insulin and tablets. Here they will control your diet and thereby reduce the need for high doses of insulin. Once you go home, your situation is the same i.e. back to square one. Many times, people do not follow   the doctor's advice and think they themselves are experts in that field.

My dear friends please follow the advice of the doctor strictly and keep a strict vigil on your diet, especially foods containing high amount of potassium, sodium, and phosphorus, so that you will save yourself from future complications. Though these are vital for us, but excess consumption will harm you.

I do not blame the doctors for this situation, it is our fault not following the doctor's advice. However, I feel they do not give you the right advice.

Another thing I have noticed is that most super specialists try to sell you high cost medicines including insulin. The reason for this is that big pharmaceutical companies, corporate hospitals, and the doctors are all hand in globe with each other. The doctors are paid incentives in various forms including cash and in kind. For example, a trip abroad, a tour in cruise vessels and so on for promoting a particular company's products. In essence, they are their brand ambassadors.

How to know what is your required daily insulin dose?

Most diabetic patients guess in the air, I mean blink, as this is the one area they do not have any idea. The doctors will never tell you how to calculate the insulin units, as it is his privilege and domain so that patients will go back to him, every now and then. I will tell you how to know your approximate insulin requirement.

This is how it is.

For example, your daily intake of food is 1800 calories; the thump rule is that one unit of insulin will reduced 50 mg/dl glucose. Therefore, your average daily insulin requirement is 1800 divided by 50=36 units/day. However, this depends upon the type of insulin prescribed by the doctor - as some are rapid acting and some are slow.

Further, most doctors prescribe twice a day insulin intake, that is, in the morning and at night. In this way, you take more units at a time and sometimes it is more and sometimes less than the required units are. In my experience, if your glucose levels are high, then it is better to take insulin thrice a day. The doctors will never tell you this unless you request them to advice that way.

However, this will depend on your food intake.

Warning

Please do not take medication into your hands and endanger your life, especially with insulin. Let the doctor do his duty and prescribe the medication as per your situation. I have just given an idea how to know the insulin requirement so that you will not take more doses than needed.

It is always better to take one or two units less initially than the prescribed daily requirement and in a few days, after checking your glucose levels with a gluco meter, you will know exactly how many units you need. As already mentioned at the beginning, in January 2013, I was sitting in my office relaxing after lunch. Suddenly I felt that my heart is beating very fast and it continued for about half an hour. I was wondering what was happening inside me. It stopped after half an hour and I was normal.

The next day I went to a cardiologist to know what has happened to me the previous day. He advised a 2D echo and ECG which revealed dilation of my Left Ventricle and Mitral Valve and given prescriptions to control the problem and advised periodical follow up to monitor the situation. Then I went to my Cardio Thoracic surgeon and he told the Valve problem does not require immediate surgery for repair or replacement, and advised to continue with the medication as I can wait. However, one thing that surprised me was that both the cardiologist and CT surgeon never advised me for a TMT or CT Angiogram except a TEE test, as I did not have any other symptoms. After one year,   around midnight, I had mild perspiration and palpitation lasting a few minutes and was normal again.

The next day I went to the Cardiologist and he told nothing to worry as I have the valve problem and advised to get a 2D Echo and ECG done, which was normal.

However, my daughter who is a Medical student asked the Cardiologist why don't you do a CT Angiogram to know whether there is any blockages. Suddenly, he looked upon her from top to bottom, and asked who she is. She told I am a doctor who completed basic Medical education. He then advised me to undergo a CT Angiogram and it revealed three blockages in my heart; one with over 90% blockage and two others with 60-70% blockages.

Based on this, he advised me to undergo an Angiogram and it revealed that I cannot do an Angioplasty or Stent insertion to open up the blockages and advised earliest Open Heart Surgery.

Then another problem cropped up as I was using a tablet for controlling my Blood Pressure. This resulted in induced throat infection with a bacteria called pseudomonas (normally found in human nose, throat and mouth), which need to be cured, as mitral valve replacement is there and this bacteria can cause severe heart infection.

However, even after several months of treatment, the condition did not improve, then the ENT specialist advised surgery, which the cardiologist objected.

Then the Cardio Vascular Surgeon along with a team of 8 doctors that consisted of few Cardiologists, an ENT specialist, a Dentist and Nephrologists, after prolonged discussions, decided to go ahead with the surgery for simultaneous bypass (CABG) and Mitral Valve replacement, stating that in any case, there is danger to my life, so better to take the risk.

The surgery went on for about nine and a half hours and after that I was in the CICU for over three days as I got my consciousness only after 75 hours. Normally, after the bypass surgery, a person gets his consciousness back within 24-36 hours, but I had complications, especially of breathing. I found out that this was due to a minor heart failure and filling of fluids in my right chest that is blood and water from the surgical wounds.

What mistake the surgeon or his team of co-surgeons and the attending technicians did was that they put only one drain bag on my left side and did not put a drain bag on my right, which resulted in breathing difficulty and I was on ventilation due to this, for almost 3 days.

They thought I may not survive as my face swelled heavily and my daughter and all relatives were informed that I was very critical. Indeed I was in a serious condition, largely, due to non draining out the fluids from my right chest. Anyway, by the grace of God, after 75 hours, I got my consciousness back and they shifted me to the Cardiac Care Unit.

I was in the hospital for 13 days and then they discharged me. The months that followed, twice I was in ICU for minor complications, and afterwards in five months I became normal. Until now, I have no major complications with the valve or bypass surgery.

After discharge from hospital, my sugar levels were quite normal and I was following their advice very strictly. However, after two years, suddenly, I felt pain in my stomach and visited a gastroenterologist surgeon, whom I know personally for many years, instead of a physician, on my own. He was a gem of a person with right knowledge and a very large heart to help the patients. He is a very popular gastro as well as general surgeon.

He prescribed some tests including an abdominal scan, after seeing the results, he came to the conclusion that I have Fatty Liver Grade one. He did not prescribe any medicines; instead, he has given a list of foods that I have to take daily to reverse the condition i.e. to reverse fatty liver to normal condition otherwise this problem can lead to Liver Cirrhosis.

Since he is a gastro surgeon, he might have read about a lot of foods that can prevent such conditions and adopted in his daily practice. This attitude makes him stand out in the crowd, and different from the herd of doctors who know everything, but never tell the patient or his attendees.

From the above experience I have become smarter and totally changed my diet habits and adopted foods as suggested by the gastro surgeon that consisted of seventy per cent vegetables in my plate, a few course of fruits and cutting down the starchy foods and carbohydrates to 20 to 30 percent of my daily intake.

This resulted in further reducing my insulin requirements and I felt happy. It is almost nine months now; I have done an abdominal scan in March 2018 to see how much reduction in the condition of Fatty Lever has taken place. Normally it takes a minimum six months to a year to reverse the condition, by strictly adopting the diet plan. The scan revealed that the condition is same and may need for time.

Special Foods for Fatty Liver

These are the foods that the gastro surgeon recommended for me to prevent fat accumulation in the liver and will help in reversing the Fatty Liver.

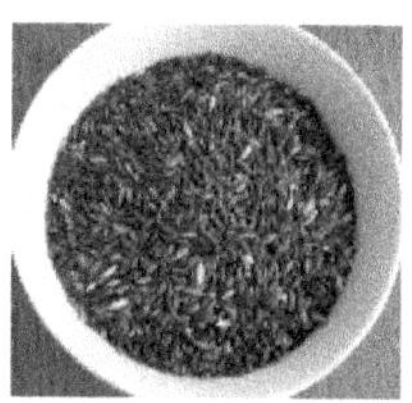

Black Rice

For one time meal, the required quantity of black rice (uncooked) is 1/3 cup or about 30-35 grams only.

To prepare the rice, soak it in water for 6-8 hours and then cook in a pressure coocker, rice cooker/induction cooker, or a small vessel including pressure pan. The ratio of rice and water is 1:3. First, cook it for five minutes in medium heat and another 10 minutes in low flame. However, direct cooking in a plain vessel, need 30-40 minutes cooking. The cooked rice will be little loose and purple in appearance, but tasty. You can powder the rice and make porridge or make any type of dish with it.

100 grams of cooked rice gives 170 calories, 34g carbohydrates, 2g dietary fiber, 5g protein, 5g total fat and no cholesterol in it. In addition, it contains many antioxidants as well.

Peruvian white Quinoa
Quinoa is a food powerhouse as it contains many important minerals, vitamins and

antioxidants. 100g cooked quinoa gives 120 calories, 26g carbohydrate, fat 3g, potassium 240 mg, dietary fiber 3g, protein 5g, no sodium, sugar, or cholesterol, and contains 10% iron, and 2% calcium.

 Chia seeds

100g cooked Chia seeds contains 480 calories, 44g carbohydrate, total fats 30g, potassium 160mg, dietary fiber 38g, protein 14g, sodium 19mg, sugar 1g, no cholesterol and iron, and 63% calcium.

No need to cook it, just soak it in water for 4-6 hours and it is ready for use. However, some people likes it cooked, then, just boil it in water for one or two minutes. Just sprinkle it in your salads, meals, milk, or snacks and consume it.

Cocoa powder (unprocessed)

100 g unprocessed cocoa powder contains 229 calories, 54g carbohydrate, fat 13g, potassium <u>1520 mg</u>, dietary fiber 33g, protein 19g, sodium 21mg, sugar 1mg, cholesterol nil, iron 77%, calcium 13%.

As cocoa is high in potassium, use a teaspoon, 5.4g, only in a day.

All kinds of vegetables viz Cucumber/ Zucchini, ash gourd/winter melon, bottle gourd, bitter gourd, snake gourd, raw bananas, red capsicum/<u>red pepper</u>. You can use any seasonal vegetables available in your region.

Foods that are a strict no for Diabetics
Fried foods including processed foods.

Sweets aerated and sweetened beverages like soft drinks (cola), soda, juice, blended coffee.

Also, avoid consuming white rice and white breads, which are full of starch and carbs. All types of Alcoholic Beverages.

Loaded or topped foods like potatoes or nachos, and dishes with rich sauces.

Fruits like sapodilla (chikoo/ supota in India), watermelon, ripe banana, and mangoes.

Chapter 5

Healthy Foods for Diabetic, Heart, and Obese Patients

Given below is a list of foods, which are good for diabetic as well as heart patients.

Whole grains (super foods) which are rich in fiber.

Black rice

Oats

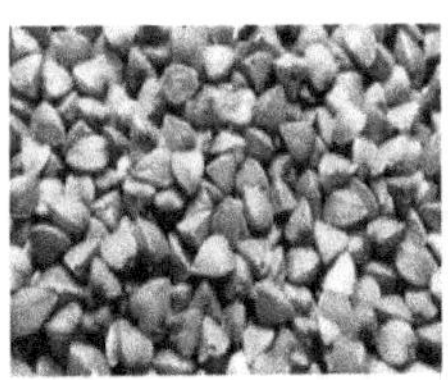

Buckwheat

Barley

Whole wheat

(Including the long grain Samba wheat in India, which contain very little starch in it).

Millets

Including finger/foxtail millet

(ragi/ bhakri/kangni/jowar/bajra, in India)

Legumes/Pulses/Lentils

Farro

Warning

Persons with cardiovascular and kidney diseases and are using medicines for high blood pressure should be very careful with food items high in potassium, phosphorus and sodium as these can endanger your life.

However, please note that most natural foods when eaten, only digests and absorbs about 40-60 percent of these items, hence need not worry about it. However, foods containing supplements and additives, especially ready to eat foods, must be avoided as it is fully absorbed i.e. 100% absorption rate.

Chapter 6

Need for Meal Planning

For meal, planning and dish ideas do a web search about different types of dishes for breakfast, lunch, dinner and in between snacks. Calorie related details, cooking methods (wiki how is a good site for cooking methods and BBC Foods for meal plans and ideas) etc can also be found this way. Select and modify the ones you like and adapt it in your daily diet. Ensure that you eat fiber rich and healthy foods, rich in proteins, minerals, and antioxidants.

A small Tip for you

Based on the type of foods you consume, prepare a list of such items, its nutritional values such as calorie, carbohydrate, potassium, phosphorus, iron, calcium, total fat, cholesterol etc, and then select the items you want on a daily basis.

For example, you consume vegetables containing more potassium in one day, but in some other day more sodium, or phosphorus, then, inter change/shuffle such items on a day-to-day basis and select the ones accordingly. This way you will maintain good intake of food without increasing potassium, phosphorus, or sodium, that is, more than the required quantity/ limit.

On an average a healthy person can consume up to 3500mg each of potassium and sodium and 700 mg of phosphorus. However, patients with kidney and heart diseases must limit potassium and sodium intake to 2000 mg/day.

For meat lovers, instead of red meat use the following - turkey or chicken breast side meat, which is less in fat.

Fish

Salmon, mackerel, tuna, or similar fishes, even tropical fishes max two or three times a week, in moderate quantity.

Boiled Egg without yoke

Fruits

Guava

Apple

Berries (all types) including gooseberry
Kiwis

Cherries

Dragon fruit

Orange

Peach/Pomegranate/ Pears

Most fruits eat half or small ones only.

Vegetables

All dark green leafy vegetables including Moringa, carrot and Amarnthus leaves. *Leafy green vegetables such as kale, spinach, and broccoli contain high amount of Vitamin K; hence, people on Warfarin must be careful.* **Amarnthus leaves are excellent source of nutrients for people who cannot afford costly items.**

Raw Pumpkin/squash - not fully ripe

Winter melon (Ash gourd)

Cucumber/zucchini

Bottle gourd

Snake gourd

Bitter gourd

Tomatoes

Raw bananas/plantain

Sweet potatoes - occasionally

Green peas

Onion

Green Beans

Cluster beans (very good for diabetics)

Egg plant, cauliflower, cabbage, and broccoli

Ladies finger/Okra (a must for diabetics)

Button mushrooms

Spices

Cinnamon

Ginger

Garlic

Turmeric

Coriander

Chilies (red/green)

Black pepper

Cumin seeds

Mustard seeds

Fenugreek seeds

The black cumin seed is very good for diabetics as it may help reduce sugar levels as well as gastric problems. Just take a few black cumin seeds, say 2-3 grams, heat it slightly, chew, and eat it.

Diabetic persons should restrict their intake of pulses / legumes / lentils, especially peanuts and green grams. Use it in limited quantity and that too occasionally as it contains high amount of proteins. If you take in large quantities, it will surge your glucose levels.

Egg users, instead of the whole egg, use boiled egg without the yellow part.

Note: All diabetic and heart patients must check the natural nutrition data of most grains/fruits and vegetables and select the items that suits you that is less in potassium, phosphorus, and sodium.

Warnings

(1) Some of the ready to eat foods viz breakfast cereals etc contains harmful additives like Butylated Hydroxytoluene (BHT), or your grilled burger may contain Monosodium Glutamate (MSG) and some foods may contain harmful ingredients like High Fructose Corn Syrup (HFCS).

Thus, it is better to use only natural products, whether it is vitamins, minerals, and other supplements, fruits, vegetables or cereals including breakfast cereals. There is no substitute for natural and homemade foods i.e. provided by nature, which are healthy and not harmful.

(2) Please, check the label before buying any readymade and packed foods that contain the above materials and/or the so-called nutrition supplements, and vitamins, not tested and approved by government authorities.

Never ever, buy these items from over the counter or from web sites selling them. Instead, buy only products that is approved, prescribed by doctors, and manufactured by reputed companies that too if it is highly essential. Otherwise, they will do more harm than good.

Meals Plan

Please remember to divide your food intake into to at least five times a day instead of the standard three meals a day. In essence, short meals (ideally every two hours) are better as you take less calories. What you can do is to take only 60 percent of your requirements during the meals and in between the meals take some light snacks, salads or soups so that you will not lose your calorie requirements.

In my experience, cooking oil is the main culprit in increasing sugar levels as it contains more unhealthy fat. Therefore, restrict oil usage to a bare minimum, the recommended use is 15 grams a day i.e. monthly 450 grams per person. Initially, it may be difficult, but when you habituate it, will become more comfortable and easy to adhere.

I am giving below a few Indian names of vegetables and grains, for those who are not familiar with English names.

All kinds of vegetables viz Cucumber (vellarika/dosa kaya/ kheera), ash gourd or winter melon i.e (poosakaya/kubalan kaya/petta), bottle gourd - kaddu/louki/sorakkaya, bitter gourd (karela/ pavakkaya/kakkara kaya), snake gourd (padavalan kaya/ chichinda), red capsicum- red pepper. Broccoli same in India, which looks like cauliflower but belongs to cauliflower family, sweet potato - ratalu/ shakarkand.

Leafy vegetables and spicy leaves: Hara dhaniya - coriander leaves, pudhina - mint leaves, Amaranths - chaulaee, cheera/ thottakura, Sarson ka patha - mustard leaves, Parsley -ajmooda in Hindi/achu moda in Kannada.

The main cause of heart vessel blockage is unhealthy fats i.e. oil, butter or margarine and fatty foods. Eliminate it or restrict it to very small quantity as suggested above, then your sugar levels will be low and chances of heart related problems will be very less.

Do not forget to include green salads in your meal plan especially with sprouted grams like chickpeas, green grams, raw carrot, cucumber, parsley, cabbage and other green leaves. You can also add a little limejuice to spice it up or use any natural vinegar (not citric acid) like apple cider vinegar, or a little coconut milk and so on.

Please use safe non-stick cookware while making dishes especially, pancakes, egg fries etc. Also, make it a habit not to use deep fried items and bakery products viz ice creams, cakes, cookies with lots of sugar. Instead of using oil-fried items like fish, steam cook or grill it, without adding starch for coverings or coatings.

Dry fruits/Nuts: Walnuts, raw Pistachios (not salted and fried) and Almonds can be taken daily or two to three times a week. However, restrict it to 5-6 pieces a day. In case you are a vegan, you can take a handful of them, in order not to lose your muscles.

Important

If you are on mechanical heart valve, remember to avoid legumes /pulses, fruits, and leafy vegetables high in Vitamin K, (Leafy green vegetables such as kale, spinach, and broccoli contain high amount of Vitamin K.).

Use of these items will result in making the Warfarin /Coumadin/ Acitrom tablets ineffective, used for keeping the blood thin and preventing clotting. However, you need not avoid these items completely, but use occasionally and in limited quantity, so that you get essential minerals and vitamins for preserving immunity and good health.

Those who use Flaxseeds, be aware that one tea spoon of flaxseeds provide 0.44 mcg of vitamin K and hence it is better to avoid it or use very rarely and that too maximum a spoon full of the seeds.

You can include fruits like papaya, banana, pineapple (not very ripe, say medium), dry grapes, grape fruits, and dates in very small quantity say 2-3 small pieces occasionally, as it will satisfy your cravings for sweets/ sugar. These fruits contain lots of important nutrients, minerals, and vitamins. Overall, ensure that your glucose level never goes beyond the normal range.

Further, you can use milk at least once a day, in the morning or at bed time. However, remember to use toned/skimmed milk rather than the fresh full cream milk. If using full cream milk, take out the cream or fat after boiling and dilute it. In addition, you can include yogurt/curd in moderate quantity but use it diluted and not very thick.

Yogurt/curd is better than milk, especially for diabetics, as it helps better digestion and prevents cravings.

Chapter 7

Reducing Sugar Levels

The key to reducing sugar levels are by reducing the starch, carbohydrate and high fat foods, especially carbohydrate intake to a max of 15-20 grams per meal and in a day 45 to 60 grams only. For this, you will have to monitor your glucose levels regularly and adjust the intake of carbs. This can be achieved through proper meal planning consisting of fruits, vegetables including sprouted legumes and whole grains/cereals, fish, egg and thin meat.

Over all, restrict your diet to the required calories, as an average person needs only 1800-2000 calories a day. However, it can vary slightly depending on the nature of your job.

Do not forget to ask your doctor or dietician to give the right diet plan for you as per your food habits and availability of items in your area and did not burden you.

By cutting down sugar, oil, salt, starch, carbohydrate, and sugar containing fruits intake, your daily insulin requirements will come down substantially.

Also, please remember, not to overcook the vegetables. As much as possible eat raw vegetables, which will reduce your craving for food and reduce problems like obesity, diabetes and other related problems viz cardio vascular diseases, kidney, liver, and eye disorders.

Cinnamon is a very effective spice which will help reduce obesity. You can add it in dishes/curries.

Perhaps it may not be possible for all to follow the information as it is, however, based on the availability of foods, and according to regional preferences, prepare a meal plan that will satisfy your taste buds, will not over burden your pocket and will help reduce the problems.

In case of doubts about certain information viz. nutritional values, cooking methods, etc., please do a web search through Google or any other browser. For detailed information consult your dietician or from authentic sites like national health boards or nutrition councils, for example USDA site ww.ndb.nal.usda.gov of US, National Institute of Nutrition, India etc. However, my sincere advices to all of you are to consult your doctor for detailed information and clarifications, regarding medication and its benefits and side effects.

Very Important

One most important thing to remember is to do regular exercises, and walking is the best, say for about 30-45 minutes daily (depending on age and health), or others like swimming, cycling, gym exercises, etc. Therefore, the key to good health is to control your diet i.e eat healthy foods rich in fiber, minerals, vitamins and antioxidants, but less in carbs and starch. Exercise well, and monitor your glucose levels regularly / periodically, as per medical advice. This will succeed only when you make it a daily habit.

I have been under the impression that my sugar levels were under control, but the sudden news of heart valve problem and following revelation of arterial blockages put me in to high alert.

However, after my bypass and valve replacement surgery, I was taking extra precautions about food and medication strictly as per medical advice. Then later on i.e. after two years I was diagnosed with fatty liver, it did not surprise me as I have been suffering from Diabetic Retinopathy for the past two years.

Now I believe that my liver problem is under control and hope nothing happens to my kidneys. So far so good and hope for the best since am taking all kinds of precautions for not to flare up things.

However to my utter surprise, when I did an abdominal ultrasound scan on 21 February,

2018 it is found that I have a Kidney stone of 3-4 mm size in my left kidney and in addition, there are several tiny stones in my gall bladder. This was due to taking several medicines especially the medicine for controlling lipids and the use of Ecosprin for a long time.

When I shown the scan report to my gastro surgeon, he suggested to remove the gallstones by laparoscopic surgery if it permits otherwise, remove the gall bladder completely by normal surgery as the stones are very small ones and may fall down from the gall bladder and can block the pancreatic tube, which will result is life-threatening situation.

On the advice of the gastro surgeon, I met my Cardiologist for his opinion and he after consulting the liver surgeon recommended that there is no need for doing anything, as the condition is asymptomatic.

Normally young persons may have severe abdominal pain and digestive disorders when gallstones are there in the gallbladder. In my case, there is no pain and no action recommended till such time I have uncontrollable pain or digestive disorders. Thank God, of now I am safe.

Along with the above test I have also got an HbA1c test and it give me a pleasant surprise that is, my A1c level has come down from 6.8 to 5.7 that means from controlled diabetes to pre-diabetic stage which is quite amazing. The main reason for the A1c level got reduced is due to my strict adherence to diet in the past five months. I hope to reduce the A1C level to 5.5 or below in the coming months. You can also reduce the A1C level to almost normal by adopting strict control on diet.

It is my earnest request to all brethrens to take care of your health by strictly following medical advice, modifying life styles and strict diet control to avoid, after effects of diabetes viz. cardiovascular diseases, eye disorders, liver, and kidney problems.

Everyone has to go when time comes, but untimely death due to diseases is the worst kind. Therefore, take care of yourself for the sake of you and your dear ones.

If you liked this book, please tell others and spread the word about it amongst your friends, relatives and your inner circle.

Thanks

About the Author

 I am a writer and author of books on general topics as well as a trained manager specializing in Sales and Marketing. However, at present am enjoying my retirement life.

My other books include Online Business - the Ultimate Success Formula, and Colo-rectal Cancer - A True Story, which are available with Create Space and Amazon Kindle.

www.ingramcontent.com/pod-product-compliance
Lightning Source LLC
Chambersburg PA
CBHW051914250726
48659CB00002B/648